Best Keto Snacks and Healthy Desserts 50+ Low Carb Snack Ideas Cookbook

By Karla Bro

Disclaimer

All material in "Best Keto Snacks and Healthy Desserts. 50+ Low Carb Snack Ideas Cookbook" is provided for your information only and may not be construed as medical advice or instruction. No action or inaction should be taken based solely on the contents of this information. Consult appropriate professionals for your health and well-being.

Remember that cooking is subjective. You may not achieve the results desired due to different brands of ingredients or different cooking abilities. Make sure you are not allergic to any ingredients.

I am not a chef. I'm just a person who likes cooking and writing about home-cooked food. Most of my recipes are created based on personal taste.

Table of Contents

Introduction

You need to eat 4-6 times a day in small portions during the ketogenic diet. But you are hungry and busy. It's not time for lunch or dinner. What can you do? Eat keto snacks!

You can use simple products in this case. We agree that often this is a good solution to the problem, and it doesn't take time for preparation.

Boiled chicken egg

You can eat one or two eggs with salt or spices. Store the product in a cold place. Therefore this variant of snack is more suitable for those who are sitting at home.

Cheese

Eat a couple of slices of favorite cheese. It can overcome hunger and replenish the stores of fats and proteins.

Ham

You can eat a few slices with lettuce leaves.

Nuts

Peanuts, walnuts, almonds, pecans and even cashews are ideal snacks. This option is fast and convenient. But remember that nuts are harmful in large quantities. Eat no more 10 pieces of nuts a day.

Seeds

You can eat seeds of sunflower or pumpkin in small quantities at work.

Avocado

Between meals you can eat half an avocado. Fruit can be salt.

Olives

It's a snack option for work or home. You can eat up to 10 pieces for one meal.

Yogurt

A cup of yogurt will satisfy hunger and give strength.

Peanut butter paste

You can eat a couple of spoons between meals. Paste must be in pure form. Any additives can saturate your body with extra carbohydrates.

Berries

You can bring half a glass of blueberries, strawberries, blackberries, raspberries or cranberries to work.

But sometimes you want to eat something else. So, we advise you use our recipes. They are useful, and some of them will only take a few min. to prepare, although others will take a few hours. Try some of these snacks in your keto system. These recipes will be useful if you are a beginner or have been on the keto system for months.

Keto Snacks

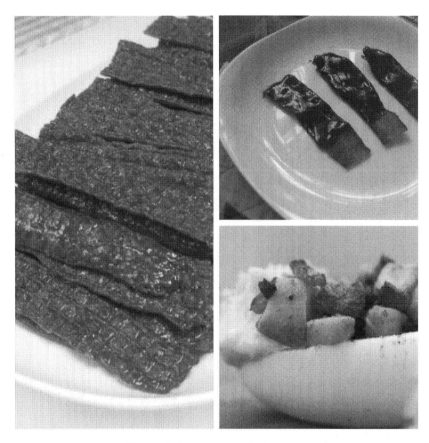

Chocolate-Covered Bacon
Caesar Deviled Eggs with Bacon and Avocado
Ground Beef Jerky

Chocolate-Covered Bacon

Ingredients

4-6 slices organic, pastured bacon, cut in half

1/2 melted block Chocolate Fuel Bar

Pink Himalayan sea salt, to taste

Cooking time: 1-2 hours

Serves: 2

Calories per person: 180

Nutritional facts: total fat 6.5g, cholesterol 10mg, sodium 390mg, total carbohydrate 22.5g, protein 8g

Directions

1. Line a baking sheet with parchment paper, and preheat your oven to 350 °F.

2. Place the bacon slices evenly on the sheet. Put the sheet in the oven.

3. Bake the bacon to crispiness, checking every 5-10 min.

4. Remove bacon from the oven. Drain away the excess fat into a jar. Use the paper towel to remove excess fat on bacon.

5. Melt the chocolate in the microwave for 30 seconds or over the stove on low heat. Poor melted

chocolate into a glass jar. Dip the bacon slices in the chocolate, covering half-way.

6. Eat immediately or place the chocolate bacon on a plate and refrigerate to allow the chocolate to harden.

7. Sprinkle with a pinch of salt, if desired.

Caesar Deviled Eggs with Bacon and Avocado

Ingredients

2 eggs

1 tbsp mayonnaise

¼ tsp Dijon mustard

Juice of 1/8 lemon

¼ tsp garlic powder

1/8 tsp Himalayan pink salt

1/8 tsp smoked paprika

¼ avocado

1 piece of pastured bacon

Cooking time: 20 min
Serves: 1
Calories per person: 411

Nutritional facts: total fat 31.6g, cholesterol 356mg, sodium 825mg, total carbohydrate 9.8g, protein 19.4g

Directions

1. Chop avocado and bacon into ¼-inch pieces.

2. Place bacon in preheated frying pan and cook over medium heat for 3 min. until brown.

3. Add avocado. Reduce heat to low. Cook for 3 minutes, stirring.

4. Boil the eggs in 2 quarts of water for 8 min.

5. Place boiled eggs in ice water for 5 min. Pell and cut eggs in half lengthwise.

6. Remove the yolks from the halved eggs. Place the yolks in a food processor, add mayonnaise, lemon juice, garlic powder, salt, and mustard. Blend the mixture until smooth.

7. Gently spoon the bacon mixture into the egg whites or use a piping bag, if desired.

Ground Beef Jerky

Ingredients

1300 g ground beef

5 tsp garlic powder

4 tsp sea salt

4 tsp fresh ground pepper

1 tbsp liquid smoke

Cooking time: 8 hours 30 min

Serves: 32 strips

Calories per person: 78

Nutritional facts: total fat 2.5g, cholesterol 36mg, sodium 261mg, total carbohydrate 0.5g, protein 12.4g

Directions

1. In a large mix bowl, mix all the ingredients.

2. Using a Jerky Gun, press 32 strips. Alternatively, use parchment paper. Roll the mixture into a thin sheet between the sheets of parchment paper. Cut into strips.

3. Place the strips on racks. Dehydrate for 7-12 hours. The beef jerky must be dry and crisp.

4. Strips can be stored in refrigerator up to 7 days.

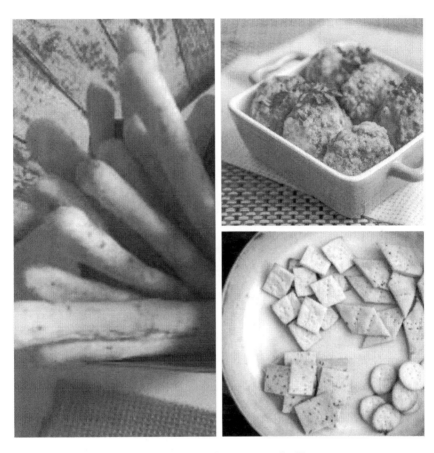

Buffalo Chicken Meatballs
Thyme Onion Crackers
Keto Breadsticks

Buffalo Chicken Meatballs

Ingredients

450 g organic chicken

1 egg, beaten

2 green onions, chopped

1 celery stalk, chopped finely

1 tbsp almond flour or coconut flour

1 tbsp organic mayonnaise

1 tsp onion powder

1 tsp garlic powder

1 tsp natural salt

1 tsp pepper

1 cup buffalo sauce for wings

Cooking time: 30 min
Serves: 4
Calories per person: 333

Nutritional facts: total fat 74.5g, cholesterol 117mg, sodium 936mg, total carbohydrate 8.2g, protein 40.3g

Directions

1. Preheat oven to 400 °F. Grease a baking sheet with coconut oil (or butter or avocado oil).

2. In a large bowl, mix all ingredients, except the buffalo sauce.

3. Make 2-inch balls from the mixture. Place the meatballs on the baking sheet. Bake for 15 min.

4. Remove the meatballs from the oven.

5. Place the meatballs in the skillet over the medium heat.

6. Add the buffalo sauce to the skillet. Cook until the sauce is warmed through.

Thyme Onion Crackers

Ingredients

1 cup sweet onion

1 large clove of garlic

¼ cup avocado oil

2 tsp fresh dried thyme

¼ tsp Himalayan salt

A pinch of fresh ground pepper

1½ cups ground flax seed

½ cup finely ground sunflower seeds

Cooking time: 2 hours 30 min.

Serves: 12

Calories per person: 119

Nutritional facts: total fat 8g, cholesterol 0mg, sodium 56mg, total carbohydrate 6.8g, protein 3.9g

Directions

1. Preheat oven to 225 °F.

2. Coarsely chop onion into 2-inch pieces.

3. Put onion, garlic, butter, salt, pepper, and thyme in a food processor. Blend until onion is mushed.

4. Add flax and sunflower seeds. Mix well.

5. Transfer the mixture to a large bowl.

6. Lay a 10-inch piece of parchment on the table. Place ½ cup of dough on the paper. Shape dough into balls and place in the middle of one side of the paper.

7. Place other piece of parchment on the dough. Roll the dough to about ¼ inch thick.

8. Remove the parchment from the dough. Cut dough into 1-inch cubes with a sharp knife.

9. Place the parchment paper with the crackers on the baking sheet. Repeat steps 6 through 8 with the remaining dough.

10. Bake crackers for 2 hours. After 1 hour, turn the crackers over and remove the paper.

11. Remove from oven and let cool on baking sheet for 15 min. Make 75 crackers.

Keto Breadsticks

Ingredients

75 g almond flour

200 g Mozzarella cheese

1 egg

3 tbsp cheese cream

1½ tsp psyllium

½ tsp baking powder

½ tsp Italian herbs

90 g Cheddar cheese

25 g Parmesan cheese

½ tsp dried garlic

2 tsp cinnamon

4 tsp erythritol

Salt and pepper, to taste

Cooking time: 30 min
Serves: 24
Calories per person: 40

Nutritional facts: total fat 2.9g, cholesterol 14mg, sodium 56mg, total carbohydrate 1.3g, protein 2.5g

Directions

1. Preheat oven to 400 °F.

2. In a medium bowl, mix the eggs and cream cheese.

3. In a separate bowl, mix the almond flour, psyllium, and baking powder.

4. Soften the Mozzarella in a microwave for 2-3 min., mixing every 15 seconds with the fork to make it soft and smooth.

5. Add the dry ingredient mixture and egg mixture to the mozzarella. Mix thoroughly.

6. Knead the dough until smooth. Form into a ball.

7. Place parchment paper on a baking tray and top with dough. Place a silicon mat on top of the dough and roll out the dough.

8. Cut the dough into 3 equal parts.

9. Sprinkle the first part with Italian herbs.

10. Sprinkle the second part with Cheddar cheese, Parmesan, and garlic.

11. Top the third part with cinnamon and sweetener.

12. Bake the breadsticks for 15 min. until crispy.

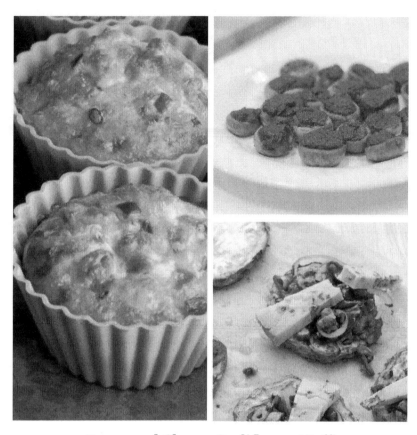

Bacon and Cheese Cauliflower Muffins
Pesto Mushrooms
Celery Root with Mushrooms and Gorgonzola

Bacon and Cheese Cauliflower Muffins

Ingredients

300 g chopped cauliflower

100 g grated Cheddar cheese

2 large chicken eggs

7 pieces bacon

25 g almond flour

25 g feta cheese

½ tsp baking powder

2 tsp garlic powder

2 tsp celery

2 tsp oregano

2 tsp paprika

Salt and pepper, to taste

Cooking time: 45 min

Serves: 12

Calories per person: 115

Nutritional facts: total fat 8.2g, cholesterol 23mg, sodium 345mg, total carbohydrate 2.7g, protein 7.9g

Directions

1. Preheat oven to 400 °F.
2. Grind the cauliflower and place in a large bowl. Add the dry ingredients, bacon, and cheese.
3. Add eggs, mix thoroughly until mixture forms.
4. Place the mixture in cupcake molds.
5. Sprinkle with feta cheese.
6. Bake for 35 min.

Pesto Mushrooms

Ingredients

200 g champignon

300 g bacon

80 g cream cheese, softened

25 g pesto with basil

Cooking time: 45 min

Serves: 5

Calories per person: 409

Nutritional facts: total fat 32.9g, cholesterol 85mg, sodium 1464mg, total carbohydrate 2.9g, protein 25.2g

Directions

1. Preheat oven to 350 °F.

2. In a bowl, mix the cream cheese with the pesto sauce.

3. Place the bacon strips on a cutting board and cut strips in half lengthwise.

4. Peel the mushrooms and remove the stems.

5. Fill each mushroom cap with the cream cheese mixture and pesto.

6. Wrap a narrow strip of bacon around each mushroom. Wind the second strip around each cap in the other direction, so the mushroom is covered with bacon.

7. Place the mushrooms on the baking sheet and put in preheated oven.

8. Bake for 20-30 min. until the bacon is crispy and a pleasant golden brown.

Celery Root with Mushrooms and Gorgonzola

Ingredients

450 g celery root

3 tbsp olive oil

100 g mushrooms

75 g spinach leaves

75 g hazelnut

3 tbsp butter

1 red onion, chopped

150 g Gorgonzola cheese

Salt and pepper, to taste

Cooking time: 50 min
Serves: 4
Calories per person: 428 calories

Nutritional facts: total fat 41.5g, cholesterol 58mg, sodium 659mg, total carbohydrate 19.1g, protein 13.6g

Directions

1. Preheat oven to 400 °F.

2. Wash and peel the celery root. Cut the root into slices or rings, 1 to 1 1/2 cm thick.

3. Smear both sides of slices with olive oil, salt, and pepper

4. Place parchment paper on the baking sheet. Put the celery on the parchment and bake in the oven for 40-45 min. until the celery becomes soft and golden.

5. Fry the mushrooms in butter until brown. Add salt and pepper.

6. Place the hazelnuts in a dry pan and fry for 5-7 min. Then, cool and chop nuts in half.

7. To make salad, mix spinach leaves, chopped red onion, mushrooms and hazelnuts in a bowl.

8. Put the salad on the cooked celery. Top with a piece of cheese and a drizzle of olive oil.

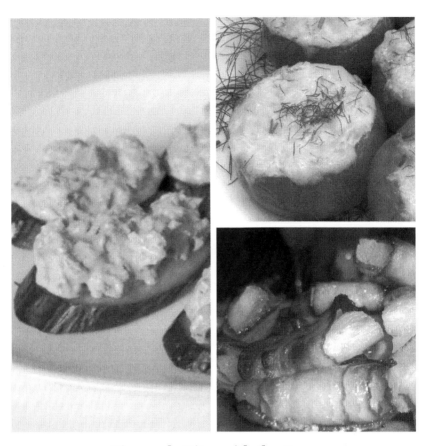

Pineapple Bites with the Bacon
Tomato Cups
California Sushi Bites

Pineapple Bites with the Bacon

Ingredients

450 g bacon slices

500 g canned pineapple chunks, drained

2 tbsp honey

¼ to ½ tsp chipotle chili powder

1 tbsp green onion, thinly sliced

Cooking time: 45 min

Serves: 20

Calories per person: 134

Nutritional facts: total fat 9.7g, cholesterol 24mg, sodium 478mg, total carbohydrate 5.7g, protein 6.6g.

Directions

1. Preheat oven to 400 °F. Line a baking sheet with foil and place a wire rack on top of the foil.

2. Cut each strip of bacon in half.

3. Weave bacon around pineapple chunks. Skewer one end of bacon strip, then pineapple.

4. Drizzle pineapple-bacon chunks with honey and chili powder.

5. Bake for 30 min. until bacon is crisp.

6. Garnish the bites with green onion to taste.

Tomato Cups

Ingredients

4 medium tomatoes

1 tbsp butter

4 eggs

2 tbsp cream

6 breakfast sausages, sliced

1 cup Cheddar cheese, shredded

2 tbsp fresh basil

salt and pepper, to taste

Cooking time: 15 min
Serves: 4
Calories per person: 169

Nutritional facts: total fat 12.4g, cholesterol 29mg, sodium 402mg, total carbohydrate 6.3g, protein 8.2g

Direction

1. Preheat oven to 350°F.

2. Cut tomatoes' tops and stems and seed tomatoes with a spoon.

3. Melt butter in frying pan over medium-low heat. Whisk eggs and cream in a medium bowl until well combined. Add salt and pepper to taste.

4. Pour egg mixture into the pan. Let sit 30 seconds without stirring. Then stir well with a wooden spoon. Cook eggs through.

5. Add sliced sausage to pan and stir. Cook 2-3 min.

6. Add half of the shredded cheese and stir. Cook 2-3 min.

7. Cool the egg mixture.

8. Fill each tomato with the mixture. Top each with remaining shredded cheese.

9. Bake 10-20 min. until tomatoes are tender and cheese is melted.

10. Top with fresh basil and serve.

California Sushi Bites

Ingredients

1 avocado

Juice of 1 lemon

1 large cucumber, sliced into 1/4" rounds

225 g lump crabmeat

1/2 cup mayonnaise

2 tsp sriracha

3 green onions, thinly sliced

Sesame seeds for garnish

Soy sauce for serving

Cooking time: 20 min
Serves: 4
Calories per person: 296

Nutritional facts: total fat 20.8g, cholesterol 64mg, sodium 518mg, total carbohydrate 15.8g, protein 13.5g

Directions

1. Peel and thinly slice avocado. Toss slices in lemon juice.

2. Top each cucumber slice with avocado. Season with salt and pepper.

3. Mix crabmeat, mayonnaise, Sriracha, and green onions in a medium bowl. Season with salt and pepper. Squeeze lemon juice onto the mixture to taste.

4. Top each cucumber slice with a small scoop of the crab mixture. Roll the slices.

5. Sprinkle sesame seeds over each serving. Serve with soy sauce.

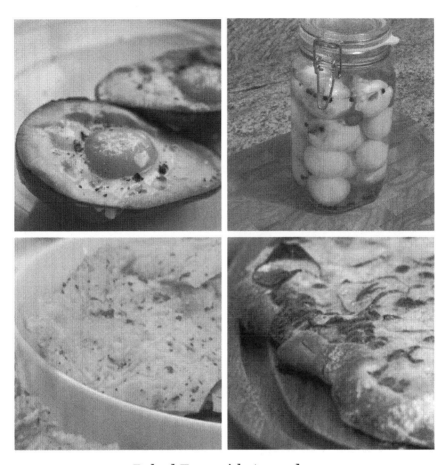

Baked Eggs with Avocado
Pickled eggs
Cheddar Taco Crisps
Keto Pizza

Baked Eggs with Avocado

Ingredients

4 eggs
2 ripe avocados
1 tsp olive oil
salt and pepper to taste

Cooking time: 20 min
Serves: 2
Calories per person: 556

Nutritional facts: total fat 50.3g, cholesterol 327mg, sodium 135mg, total carbohydrate 18g, protein 14.9g

Directions

1. Preheat oven to 350°F. Coat a baking sheet with oil.

2. Cut the avocado in half and remove the seed. Remove 2 tsp of pulp, making a hollow for the egg in the avocado.

3. Break the egg. Pour it into the avocado. Add salt and pepper.

4. Place the avocado on the baking sheet.

5. Bake for 15 min. For more well-done eggs, increase baking time.

Pickled eggs

Ingredients

12 eggs

1 cup white vinegar

½ cup water

2 tbsp coarse salt

2 tbsp pickling spice

1 sliced onion

5 black peppercorns

Cooking time: 3 days 35 min

Serves: 12

Calories per person: 78

Nutritional facts: total fat 4,4g, cholesterol 164mg, sodium 1023mg, total carbohydrate 1,6g, protein 5,6g

Directions

1. Boil the eggs. Cool them in cold water, then peel and place into a 1-quart wide-mouth jar.

2. Combine the vinegar, salt, water, pickling spice, onion (reserving a couple of slices), and black peppercorns in a saucepan. Boil the mixture for 10 min.

3. Pour the mixture into the jar. Top with the slices of onion. Seal the jar.

4. Cool the eggs. Refrigerate for 3 days before eating.

Cheddar Taco Crisps

Ingredients

¾ cup full-fat Cheddar, finely shredded

¼ cup Parmesan, shredded

¼ tsp chili powder

1/4 tsp ground cumin

Large pinch of cayenne pepper

Cooking time: 15 min

Serves: 5-6

Calories per person: 88

Nutritional facts: total fat 6.7g, cholesterol 22mg, sodium 176mg, total carbohydrate 0.6g, protein 6.6g

Directions

1. Preheat oven to 400 ˚F.

2. Line a baking sheet with a silicone baking mat.

3. Mix the Cheddar, Parmesan, chili powder, cumin, and cayenne in a small bowl.

4. Place heaping tablespoonfuls of the cheese mixture on the baking sheet 1 inch apart.

5. Spread out each pile, and pat down lightly.

6. Cook about 5 min. Bake until the cheese is golden brown and bubbly.

7. Let the crisps cool for a few seconds on the baking sheet.

8. Using a metal spatula, lift and drape the crisps over a rolling pin to cool completely.

9. Eat or store in an airtight container at room temperature for about 2 days.

Keto Pizza

Ingredients

<u>Sauce</u>

1/3 cup canned sugar-free crushed tomatoes

1 tsp olive oil

1 small clove garlic, minced

A pinch of kosher salt

<u>Keto Dough</u>

1 ½ cups shredded Mozzarella

2 tbsp full-fat sour cream

2/3 cup almond flour

2 large eggs, lightly beaten

A pinch of kosher salt

Olive oil

<u>Toppings</u>

1/3 cup shredded whole-milk Mozzarella

Crushed red pepper flakes and dried oregano, for sprinkling

Cooking time: 1 hours
Serves: 6-8
Calories per person: 160

Nutritional facts: total fat 4,5g, cholesterol 51mg, sodium 86mg, total carbohydrate 1,2g, protein 3,8g

Directions

Sauce

1. Combine the tomatoes, minced garlic, and salt in a small bowl.

2. Let the mixture sit for 30 min. at room temperature.

Dough

1. Place the cheese and sour cream in a large microwave-safe bowl.

2. Microwave the ingredients in one-minute intervals, stirring until the cheese is melted. Cool the mixture slightly.

3. Add the eggs, flour, and ¼ tsp of salt to the cheese mixture. Mix with your hands until a stretchy, slightly wet dough forms.

Pizza

1. Adjust an oven rack to the low position and place a baking sheet on it.

2. Preheat oven to 450 °F.

3. Grease a piece of parchment paper with olive oil.

4. Lightly coat your hands in oil and place the dough on the parchment, patting into a ¼-inch-thick

rectangle. Make the edges a bit thicker to create a crust all around.

5. Place the dough on the baking sheet. Bake until puffy and golden. Cook about 15 min.

6. Remove the dough from the oven and top with sauce and mozzarella. Bake pizza until it's heated through and cheese is melted, about 5 min.

7. Remove the dough from the oven.

8. Sprinkle with pepper flakes, salt, and oregano.

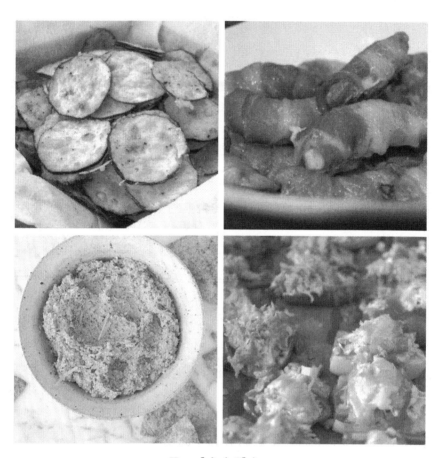

Zucchini Chips
Spicy Edamame Dip
Bacon Shrimp and Scallops
Keto Bell Pepper Nachos

Zucchini Chips

Ingredients

1 small zucchini

Cooking spray

Salt

Cooking time: 1 hour 20 min

Serves: 4

Calories per person: 5

Nutritional facts: total fat 0.1g, cholesterol 0mg, sodium 3mg, total carbohydrate 1g, protein 0.4g

Directions

1.   Line a baking sheet with a silicone mat and generously coat with cooking spray.

2.   Slice the zucchini 1/16- to 1/8-inch thick, using a mandolin.

3.   Arrange the slices on the baking sheet in a single layer.

4.   Coat with cooking spray and sprinkle with salt.

5.   Bake at 250 °F for 50 min.

6.   Flip the slices. Bake until browned about 30 min.

7.   Remove the baking sheet from the oven. Transfer the chips to a rack to cool.

Spicy Edamame Dip

Ingredients

8 cups water

4 large unpeeled garlic cloves

450 g shelled edamame beans

½ tsp cayenne pepper

¼ tsp ground cumin

4 tbsp olive oil

¼ cup fresh lime juice

¼ cup fresh cilantro, finely chopped

Pinch of salt and pepper

Pita chips for dipping

Cooking time: 45 min
Serves: 10
Calories per person: 123

Nutritional facts: total fat 8.2g, cholesterol 0mg, sodium 190mg, total carbohydrate 7.8g, protein 5g

Directions

1. Heat a medium frying pan over medium heat. Roast the garlic, turning frequently, until light brown, for 15 min.

2. Remove the garlic from the pan. Cool and peel. Set aside.

3. Boil water in a saucepan. Add beans and return to a boil. Cook for 5 min. Before draining, reserve ¾ cup of cooking water.

4. Drain the beans and cool.

5. Place the garlic into the food processor and coarsely chop.

6. Add the beans, cumin, salt, and cayenne pepper and combine.

7. Add the olive oil, lime juice, and cilantro. Combine again.

8. Add the reserved water a little at a time and combine until smooth.

9. Use pita chips for dipping.

Bacon Shrimp and Scallops

Ingredients

12 jumbo raw shrimp, peeled and deveined

12 large sea scallops, trimmed and well-drained

1 lime

1 tbsp toasted sesame oil

1 tbsp salt and black pepper

1 tsp hot red pepper flakes

12 slices smoked bacon, cut in half

Toothpicks

3 scallions, thinly sliced on an angle

Cooking time: 26 min
Serves: 12
Calories per person: 292

Nutritional facts: total fat 13.2g, cholesterol 201mg, sodium 680mg, total carbohydrate 4.7g, protein 35.5g

Directions

1. Preheat oven to 425 °F.

2. Place shrimp and scallops in a bowl and dress with lime juice and zest. Generously drizzle sesame oil over shrimp and scallops. Add salt and hot pepper flakes.

3. Wrap each shrimp and scallop with a half slice of bacon and fasten bacon in place with toothpicks. Wrap each shrimp from head to tail, and wrap the bacon around the outside of each scallop.

4. Place the shrimp and scallops on a boiler pan, for comfort, draining while bacon crisps. Bake for 10 to 14 min. Shrimp must be pink and curled, while scallops should be opaque and bacon crisp.

5. Place seafood on a dish and sprinkle with chopped scallions.

Keto Bell Pepper Nachos

Ingredients

2 medium bell peppers

1 tbsp vegetable oil

¼ tsp chili powder

¼ tsp ground cumin

120 g ground beef

1 cup full-fat shredded Mexican blend cheese

¼ cup guacamole

¼ cup Pico de Gallo

2 tbsp full-fat sour cream

Kosher salt

Cooking time: 25 min
Serves: 4
Calories per person: 260

Nutritional facts: total fat 10,7g, cholesterol 33mg, sodium 187mg, total carbohydrate 6,2g, protein 12,2g

Directions

1.   Cut the bell peppers into sixths. Remove the stem and seeds.

2.   Transfer the slices to a large microwave safe bowl. Add a splash of water and a pinch of salt. Cover

the bowl and microwave about 4 min. until the pieces are pliable.

3. Cool slightly. Line a baking sheet with the foil. Arrange the slices close together on the baking sheet.

4. Heat the oil in a large nonstick skillet over medium-high heat.

5. Add the chili powder and cumin. Cook, stirring, for about 30 seconds.

6. Add the ground beef and ¼ tsp salt. Cook, stirring until browned and cooked through, about 4 min.

7. Preheat the broiler to 425 °F.

8. Spoon some beef mixture onto each pepper piece. Sprinkle the pieces with cheese, and bake for 1 minute, until the cheese melts.

9. Top with dollops of guacamole and Pico de Gallo.

10. Mix the sour cream with a little water. Drizzle the mixture over the nachos.

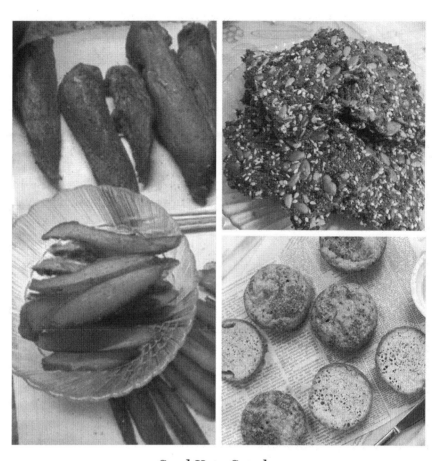

Seed Keto Snacks
Dried Chicken Breast a la "Carpaccio"
Buns with Oregano

Seed Keto Snacks

Ingredients

30 g brown flax

30 g chia seeds

30 g poppy seeds

30 g sesame seeds

30 g black sesame seeds

30 g almond flour

15 g cedar oil

240 g water

30 g pumpkin seeds

Cooking time: 50 min

Serves: 4

Calories: 352.8

Nutritional facts: total fat 30.1g, total carbohydrate 10.8g, protein 11.2g

Directions

1. Preheat oven to 300 °F
2. Bring water to a boil in a medium pan.
3. Mix dry ingredients in a separate bowl. Pour boiling water and oil over the dry mixture. Mix the ingredients.

4. Line a baking sheet with parchment paper. Place the seed dough on the paper, and top with another piece of paper. Roll the dough out flat.
5. Remove the paper from the top of the dough. Place the baking sheet in the oven. Bake about 45 min.

Dried Chicken Breast a la "Carpaccio"

Ingredients

1 kg chicken breast

5 tsp salt

2 tsp coriander

1/2 tsp spices, to taste

1 tsp black pepper

3 tsp sweet pepper

Paprika

Cooking time: 6 h 10 min
Serves: 4
Calories per person: 315

Nutritional facts: total fat 6,6g, cholesterol 160mg, sodium 3037mg, total carbohydrate 7,5g, protein 54g

Directions

1. Cut each half of a chilled breast lengthwise into two parts. You'll have 4 long thick pieces.

2. Pat each piece dry with a paper towel.

3. Mix the spices and crush before drying chicken.

4. Roll each chicken piece in spices until well coated and salt lightly.

5. Put the chicken in a container, pressing the pieces down.

6. Place the container in the refrigerator for 6-8 hours.

6. After cooling cut a small piece of rinse and taste. Taste a small piece of chicken to see if it is too salty. If it's not too salty, rinse the chicken under water. If it is salty, soak the chicken for 30 min. before rinsing. Then, rinse again and dry.

7. Cut the chicken into pieces, cover pieces in paprika. Then, string pieces on skewers for kebabs. Hang these skewers to dry at room temperature for 12-16 hours.

Buns with Oregano

Ingredients

4 eggs

4 tbsp olive oil

50 g almond flour

¼ tsp salt

1 tbsp dried oregano

Cooking time: 30 min

Serves: 6

Calories per person: 131

Nutritional facts: total fat 11g, total carbohydrate 1g, protein 7g

Directions

1. Preheat oven to 390 ºF.

2. Thoroughly mix the eggs, olive oil, flour, ¾ of the oregano, and the salt.

3. Pour the mixture into a 6-cup muffin mold.

4. Sprinkle with the remaining oregano.

5. Bake for 25 min. Then, cool at room temperature before removing the buns from molds.

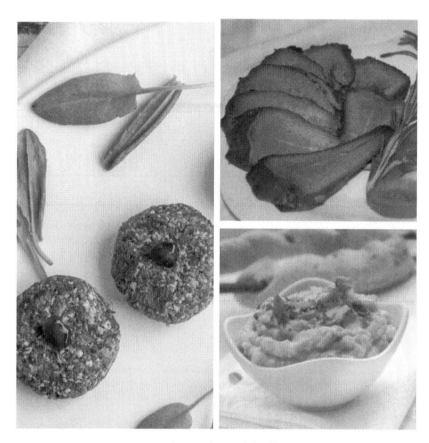

Georgian Pkhali
Pig Tongue
Eggplant Estragon Cream

Georgian Pkhali

Ingredients

1 cup walnuts

1 bunch spinach, roughly chopped

1 bunch parsley, roughly chopped

2 cloves garlic, peeled

½ tsp salt

Lemon juice to taste

Cooking time: 2 hours 15 min.
Serves: 3
Calories: 288

Nutritional facts: total fat 25g, cholesterol 0mg, sodium 480mg, total carbohydrate 9.1g, protein 13.5g

Directions

1. Soak the nuts in water for at least 2 hours.

2. Drain and rinse the nuts, then blend in a food processor.

3. Peel the garlic.

4. Cut the greens.

5. Add garlic and greens. Blend until a homogeneous mixture forms.

6. Add lemon juice and salt to taste.
7. Roll into medium balls.

Pig Tongue

Ingredients

1 800-gram pig tongue

1 stick cinnamon

2 pieces badian

5 peppercorns black pepper

2 bay leaves

1 pinch of chili pepper

1 clove garlic

30 g celery root

3-4 pinches of salt

For cranberry sauce

200 g cranberries, fresh or frozen

2 tsp sugar

1 pinch of salt

30 ml water

Cooking time: 50 min
Serves: 6
Calories: 712

Nutritional facts: total fat 46.7g, cholesterol 365mg, sodium 356mg, total carbohydrate 7g, protein 60.6g

Directions

1. Wash the pork tongue and place in a saucepan. Cover with water, add the spices, and bring to a boil.

2. Boil on a medium heat for 35-40 min.

3. Remove from the heat. Rinse the tongue with cold water and peel.

4. Place the cranberries in saucepan. Add sugar, salt, and water.

5. Cook the ingredients on medium heat for 15 min.

6. Sieve the cranberry mass. If the sauce is too thin, reduce over low heat.

7. Cut pork tongue into thin slices, serve on a plate with cranberry sauce on top.

Eggplant Estragon Cream

Ingredients

600 g eggplant

10 g chili pepper

10 g estragon (leaves)

100 g cream cheese

salt to taste

Cooking time: 35 min

Serves: 2

Calories: 275

Nutritional facts: total fat 18.5g, cholesterol 55mg, sodium 238mg, total carbohydrate 24g, protein 7.9g

Directions

1.   Preheat oven to 390 °F.

2.   Wash the eggplants. Then, cut in half lengthwise.

3.   Place eggplant on a baking sheet. Sprinkle with olive oil. Bake for 25 min.

4.   Remove the eggplants from the oven. Cool on a plate before peeling.

5.   Put the baked eggplants in the bowl of a blender.

6.   Add estragon, chili pepper, and cream cheese. Blend until smooth.

7.   Salt to taste.

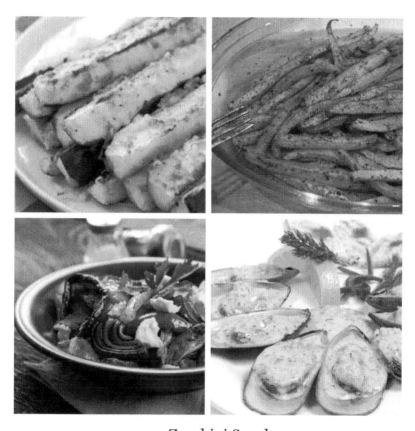

Zucchini Snack
Rosemary Carrot
Vegetable with Cheese

Zucchini Snack

Ingredients

400 g zucchini

½ tsp dry ground hot pepper

1 tbsp ground paprika

2 tbsp olive oil

Salt (to taste)

Cooking time: 15 min.   Serves: 2
Calories: 162

Nutritional facts: total fat 14.8g, cholesterol 0mg, sodium 99mg, total carbohydrate 8.7g, protein 3g

Directions

1. Preheat oven to 390 °F.

2. Wash and cut the zucchini into small squares. Put squares in a bowl.

3. Add salt, paprika, hot pepper, and olive oil to the bowl. Mix well.

4. Line a baking sheet with parchment paper. Put zucchini squares on the sheet and bake for 10 min.

Rosemary Carrot

Ingredients

300 g baby carrots

2 sprigs of rosemary, leaves only

1 pinch of sea salt

20 g butter

1 tbsp olive oil

Cooking time: 15 min

Serves: 2

Calories: 186

Nutritional facts: total fat 15.4g, cholesterol 22mg, sodium 292mg, total carbohydrate 12.8g, protein 1.1g

Directions

1. Wash the carrots. Do not remove green tails from the tops.

2. In a non-stick pan, heat the butter and add olive oil. Place the carrots in the pan. Fry until light brown on all sides.

3. Add the sprigs of rosemary. Continue frying for a few min.

4. Place carrots on a plate and sprinkle with sea salt to taste.

Vegetable with Cheese

Ingredients

200 g celery stalks

200 g carrot

200 g zucchini

200 g eggplant

200 g Dorblu cheese

2 tbsp olive oil

250 g sour cream

Salt, to taste

mint leaves or cilantro

Cooking time: 15-50 min
Serves: 4
Calories: 445

Nutritional facts: total fat 37g, cholesterol 80mg, sodium 464mg, total carbohydrate 14.6g, protein 16.4g

Directions

1. Preheat oven to 350 °F.

2. Wash the vegetables and peel the carrots. Chop everything into large strips.

3. Cut celery stalks into small pieces.

4. Cover a baking sheet with parchment paper.

5. Arrange the vegetables on the baking sheet.

6. Top the vegetables with chopped cheese. Pour olive oil over the ingredients. Sprinkle with a pinch of salt.

7. Bake in the oven for 15-50 min. If you like crispy vegetables, cook for 15-20 min.

8. Remove from the oven. Let cool slightly and serve with a sauce.

Sauce

1. Mix sour cream, crushed cilantro or mint leaves, and a pinch of salt.

Cream Mussels with Blue Cheese

Ingredients

500-600 g mussels in the shells, fresh or frozen

80-100 g Dorblu Cheese

juice of ½ orange

100-150 ml cream, 33% fat

2 tbsp mustard with grains

2 tbsp hot chili sauce

Cooking time: 10-15 min

Serves: 2

Calories: 523

Nutritional facts: total fat 21.8g, cholesterol 119mg, sodium 2185mg, total carbohydrate 19.2g, protein 61 g

Directions

1. For fresh mussels, wash the mussels and remove the "beards" attached to the shells.

2. For frozen mussels, defrost. As a rule, these have already been cleaned.

3. Preheat oven to 350 °F. Put the mussels on a large baking sheet or in a deep pan.

4. Put a small piece of Dorblu cheese in each shell with mussel and cover them with cream.

5. Mix the mustard and orange juice. Top the shells with this mixture.

6. Bake in the oven for 10-15 min.

7. Remove from the oven, arrange the mussels on a plate, and add a little hot chili sauce to each mussel or sprinkle with a small amount of chili flakes.

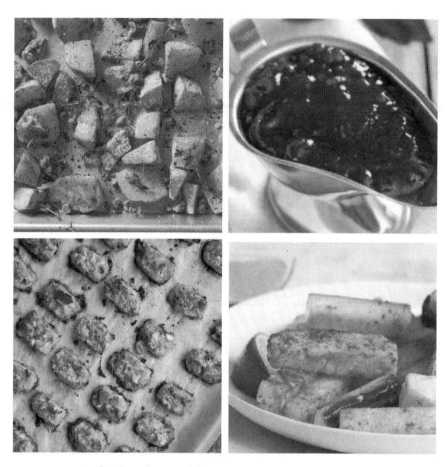

Baked Celery with Berry Sauce(top 1+2)
Cheesy Cauliflower Tots
Chili-Lime Pineapple Cucumber Sticks

Baked Celery with Berry Sauce

Ingredients

300 g celery root

100 g cream cheese

100 g black currant, fresh or frozen

1 sprig of red basil

1 sprig mint

1 tbsp olive oil

Salt and pepper, to taste

Cooking time: 35 min
Serves: 2
Calories: 331

Nutritional facts: total fat 24.7g, cholesterol 55mg, sodium 281mg, total carbohydrate 24.5g, protein 4.8g

Directions

Celery

1. Preheat oven to 350 °F.

2. Wash and peel the celery. Cut into 5-mm thick slices.

3. Cover a baking sheet with parchment paper. Place the celery slices on the baking sheet. Pour olive oil over the celery.

4. Bake for 30 min., until celery is soft.

Sauce

1. Place the berries and sugar in a medium pan. Boil for 10 min. over medium heat.

2. If mixture becomes too thick, add water.

3. Remove the berries from the heat. Wipe and sieve them.

4. Mix cream cheese into berries mixture until smooth.

5. Serve baked celery with berry sauce, mint leaves, and basil.

6. Add coarse salt and freshly ground pepper to taste.

Cheesy Cauliflower Tots

Ingredients

800 g cauliflower

1/4 cup avocado oil

1 large egg

1 ½ cup Mozzarella

2 cloves garlic, minced

¾ tsp sea salt

Cooking time: 20 min

Serves: 8

Calories per person: 59

Nutritional facts: total fat 2.6g, cholesterol 26mg, sodium 247 mg, total carbohydrate 6.2g, protein 4.4g

Directions

1. Grate the cauliflower into rice-sized pieces. Add 2 tbsp oil to a large frying pan.

2. Add the cauliflower and stir fry over medium-high heat until soft and lightly brown.

3. Whisk the egg in a large bowl. Add the mozzarella, garlic, and sea salt. Mix well.

4. Add hot riced cauliflower to the egg mixture. The cheese will melt, making the mixture sticky.

5. Using a small cookie scoop, pick up balls of mixture and flatten slightly.

6. Wipe the pan with a paper towel lightly to get rid of any cauliflower rice pieces.

7. Heat the remaining 2 tbsp avocado oil in the pan over medium heat. Add the balls in a single layer. Fry for about 2 minutes, until golden on the bottom. Flip and fry until golden on the other side.

8. Transfer to paper towels to drain.

Chili-Lime Pineapple Cucumber Sticks

Ingredients

5 spears jicama

5 spears pineapple

5 spears cucumber

1 tsp chili lime seasoning

2 lime wedges

Cooking time: 30 min

Serves: 3

Calories: 70

Nutritional facts: total fat 0g, cholesterol 0mg, sodium 261mg, total carbohydrate 15.2g, protein 0.4g

Directions

1. Cut jicama, pineapple, cucumber, and chili into strips and place strips in a bowl.

2. Add lime seasoning and lime juice to the strips. Combine the ingredients.

3. Place the strips in a resealable bag. Mix the ingredients again.

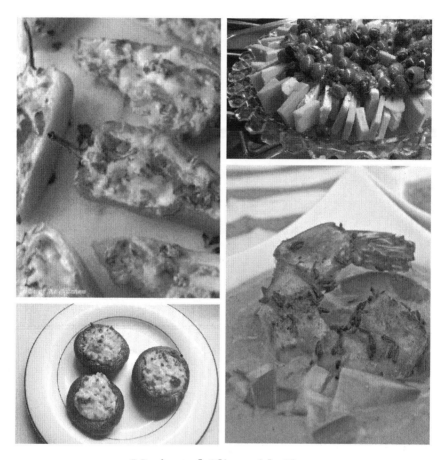

Marinated Olive with Cheese
Stuffed Mushrooms with Sausage
Stuffed Cheese Bell Pepper
Grilled Shrimp and Avocado

Marinated Olive with Cheese

Ingredients

225 g cream cheese, cold

300 g sharp white Cheddar cheese

1/3 cup pimiento-stuffed olives

1/3 cup pitted Greek olives

1/4 cup balsamic vinegar

1/4 cup olive oil

1 tbsp fresh parsley, minced

1 tbsp fresh basil, minced

2 garlic cloves, minced

60 g canned pimiento strips, drained and chopped

Cooking time: 8 hours 25 min
Serves: 16
Calories: 168

Nutritional facts: total fat 16g, cholesterol 34mg, sodium 260mg, total carbohydrate 2g, protein 6g

Directions

1. Cut the cheese in half lengthwise. Cut each half into 1/4-inch slices.

2. Arrange cheeses upright in a ring on a serving plate. Alternate cheddar and cream cheese slices.

3. Place olives in the center of the plate.

4. Whisk vinegar, oil, parsley, basil, and garlic in a small bowl until blended

5. Drizzle the seasoning over olives and cheese.

6. Sprinkle the ingredients with the pimientos.

7. Cool at least 8 hours or overnight in the refrigerator.

Stuffed Mushrooms with Sausage

Ingredients

20-24 large mushrooms

450 g Italian sausage, sliced

1 onion

330 g grated Parmesan cheese

¼ cup Italian bread crumbs

1 tsp minced garlic

1 tsp chopped fresh parsley

Cooking time: 45 min

Serves: 12

Calories per person: 238

Nutritional facts: total fat 16.8g, cholesterol 51mg, sodium 577mg, total carbohydrate 5g, protein 17.9g

Directions

1. Preheat oven to 350 °F.

2. Hollow out mushroom caps, save scrapings.

3. Heat frying pan over medium-high heat. Add sausage, onion, and reserved mushroom scrapings.

Cook and stir the ingredients 4-6 minutes until sausage is browned.

4. Drain and discard liquid. And fry again.

5. Add 330g Parmesan cheese, bread crumbs, garlic, and parsley to sausage mixture. Cook 3-5 min.

6. Cool sausage mixture. Stuff each mushroom cap with mixture. Place the stuffed caps on a baking sheet. Bake for 12 minutes. Then sprinkle remaining 120g Parmesan cheese over mushrooms. Bake until cheese is melted and bubbling, about 3 min.

Stuffed Cheese Bell Pepper

Ingredients

2 bell peppers, 300 g

2 chicken eggs

½ cup mozzarella cheese

½ cup Parmesan cheese

½ cup ricotta cheese

3 tbsp dried parsley

1 cup spinach

salt

Cooking time: 45 min

Serves: 4

Calories per person: 166

Nutritional facts: total fat 9.1g, cholesterol 91mg, sodium 275mg, total carbohydrate 9.8g, protein 12.7g

Directions

1. Preheat the oven to 370 ºF.

2. Wash and peel the peppers. Cut them in half lengthwise.

3. Mix cheese, eggs, and dried parsley in a blender.

4. Stuff each half with cheese mixture.

5. Put spinach on the top of the pepper. Bake for 30 min.

6. Sprinkle the Parmesan on the peppers and return to the oven for 5 min.

Grilled Shrimp and Avocado

Ingredients

450 g shrimp (16 shrimp)

½ tsp salt

1 tsp black pepper

1 tbsp onion powder

1 lemon

2 tbsp coconut aminos

2 tbsp avocado oil

2 ripe avocados

Cooking time: 15 min

Serves: 8

Calories per person: 152

Nutritional facts: total fat 8.7g, cholesterol 118mg, sodium 290mg, total carbohydrate 4.1g, protein 13.8g

Directions

1. Peel and clean the shrimps. Place them in a bowl.

2. Add salt, coconut aminos, pepper, onion powder. Add the juice of one half of the lemon. Combine.

3. Heat the grill or frying pan. Add avocado oil. Place shrimp in pan and cook for 3 min. Flip the shrimp.

4. Remove the shrimp and cool.

5. Peel and mush avocado with the fork. Add a little salt and lemon juice.

6. Put avocado mixture and the shrimp on the plate

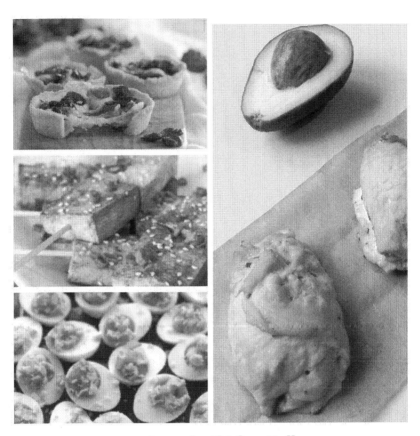

Avocado Chicken Roll
Savory Bacon Cranberry Cheese Tartlets
Buffalo Deviled Eggs
Tofu Skewers and Walnut Pesto

Avocado Chicken Roll

Ingredients

100 g fried chicken breast

1 tbsp mayonnaise

½ medium avocado, 75 g

salt

pepper

Cooking time: 15 min

Serves: 1

Calories per person: 450

Nutritional facts: total fat 29.2g, cholesterol 95mg, sodium 345mg, total carbohydrate 12.7g, protein 35.5g

Directions

1. Cut the chicken into thin long strips.

2. Cut avocado into medium slices, put them in a plate, mix with mayonnaise and salt and pepper to taste.

3. Put avocado mixture on the meat strips. Roll strips.

Savory Bacon Cranberry Cheese Tartlets

Ingredients

Tart crust

2 cups blanched almond flour

1 egg

⅓ cup butter melted

⅛ tsp sea salt

Filling

6 chopped bacon slices

1 ½ cups cubed Mahon Menorca Semi-Cured Cheese

½ cup unsweetened dried cranberries

1 tbsp fresh thyme leaves

⅛ tsp salt

⅛ tsp black pepper to taste

Cooking time: 40 min

Serves: 12

Calories per person: 158

Nutritional facts: total fat 26g, cholesterol 83mg, sodium 800mg, total carbohydrate 8g, protein 19g

Directions

1. Preheat oven to 370 °F. Grease 12-cup muffin pan.

2. Combine the ingredients for the crust. Form dough.

3. Make 12 balls with your hands. Place one into each cup.

4. Press dough with a small glass to make the tart crusts.

5. Bake the crusts for 7 min. until lightly golden. Remove them from the oven.

6. Fill the crusts with fried and chopped bacon, cubed Mahon Menorca cheese, and dried cranberries.

7. Sprinkle the tartlets with salt, pepper, and fresh thyme leaves.

8. Bake for 10 min. or until cheese is completely melted.

9. Remove the tartlets and cool for 10 minutes.

Buffalo Deviled Eggs

Ingredients

6 hard boiled chicken eggs, large

170 g boiled and chopped chicken

¼ onion

¼ cup blue cheese crumbles

¼ cup Franks Buffalo Wing Sauce

1 small chopped celery

2 tbsp blue cheese dressing

Cooking time: 20 min

Serves: 6

Calories per person: 152

Nutritional facts: total fat 12g, cholesterol 239mg, sodium 283mg, total carbohydrate 2g, protein 29g

Directions

1. Boil the eggs.

2. Chop the chicken and celery.

3. Peel cooked and cooled eggs. Cut them in half lengthwise. Separate the yolks from the egg whites and place yolks in mixing bowl.

4. Add chicken, celery, blue cheese, Franks Buffalo Wing Sauce and dressing to yolks.

5. Press the onion and add juice to the bowl. Mix all the ingredients.

6. Stuff the egg whites with yolk mixture using a fork or spoon. You can also pipe the yolks into the whites using a Ziploc bag with the tip cut off.

Tofu Skewers and Walnut Pesto

Ingredients

<u>Tofu Skewers</u>

1 kg firm tofu

2 garlic cloves

3 tbsp soy sauce

3 tbsp rice wine vinegar

1 egg white

1/3 cup sesame seeds

Wood skewers

<u>Walnut Pesto</u>

1 cup walnut pieces

1 cup fresh basil

½ cup parsley

¾ tsp salt

1 minced garlic clove

1 tsp minced ginger

1/3 cup olive oil

1 orange, zest, and juice

Cooking time: 30 min + time for chilling
Serves: 4
Calories per person: 652

Nutritional facts: total fat 53g, cholesterol 24mg, sodium 1183mg, total carbohydrate 18g, protein 38g

Directions

1. Cut tofu into 12 lengths. Skewer each piece with a wooden skewer.

2. Whisk garlic, soy, and rice vinegar in a bowl. Coat tofu with this mixture. Chill tofu from 1 to 6 hours.

3. Preheat the oven to 400 °F. Place parchment paper on a baking sheet.

4. Whisk egg white well.

5. Put tofu in the marinade.

6. Brush skewers with egg white.

7. Sprinkle tofu with sesame seeds. Place the lengths on a sheet. Bake 5 min. Turn skewers over, bake 5 minutes more.

Cooking Walnut Pesto

1. Place walnut pieces in a sauté pan. Cook for 5 min. until browned slightly.

2. Cool the walnuts.

3. Place walnut pieces, basil, salt, parsley, garlic, zest and juice of an orange, and ginger in the bowl of a food processor. Mix the ingredients.

4. Add olive oil and mix briefly.

5. Chill pesto.

Keto Sweet Snacks - Desserts

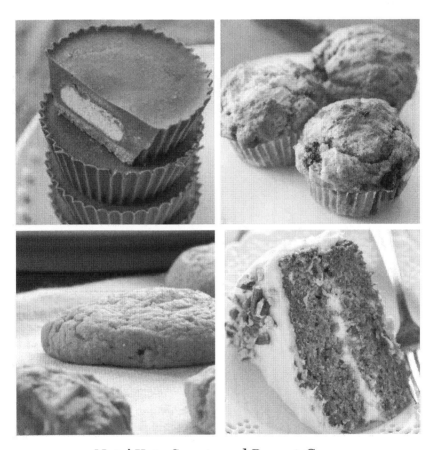

Nuts' Keto Sweets and Peanut-Cream
Nuts and Berries Cupcakes
Almond Cookies
Carrot Nut Cake

Nuts' Keto Sweets and Peanut-Cream

Ingredients

0.5 cup coconut oil

1 tbsp cocoa powder

0.5 tsp sweetener

vanilla

almonds, walnuts, peanuts, and/or hazelnuts

peanut paste to taste

butter to taste

Cooking time: 2 h 15 min

Serves: 2-4

Calories per person: 264-527

Nutritional facts: total fat 29g, cholesterol 0mg, sodium 34mg, total carbohydrate 2,4g, protein 1g

Directions

1. Prepare a water bath. Melt coconut oil, but do not overheat.

2. Add cocoa and sweetener to melted oil. Add vanilla to taste. Stir. You can change the number of

ingredients if you want. Pour half the contents into molds.

3. Put the nut or peanut-cream filling in each candy. Cover with rest of coconut oil mixture and sprinkle cocoa powder on the sweets with nuts immediately. Place in the refrigerator to harden.

4. Wait for the bottom layer of the candy to cool before stuffing. Mix 100 g of paste and 30 g of oil (or your choice). Add to the thickened bottom layer of chocolates. Then cover with the second part of the mixture.

5. Put the candy in the fridge. Keep the keto-candies in the cold.

Nuts and Berries Cupcakes

Ingredients

100 g peanut butter without any flavoring

30 g cocoa powder

1 chicken egg

1/4 tsp. soda

1/4 tsp vinegar

salt

walnuts, almonds, hazelnuts, and/or pecans (50 g for each kind)

dried or fresh berries (blueberries or cranberries)

Cooking time: 30 min
Serves: 4-6
Calories per person: 200-300

Nutritional facts: total fat 23g, cholesterol 0mg, sodium 108mg, total carbohydrate 20g, protein 11g

Directions

1. Preheat oven to 345 °F.

2. In a deep container, place the peanut butter and cocoa powder. Add egg and beat. Add soda, vinegar, and salt. Mix the ingredients using a blender to make a uniform creamy mass.

3. Add nuts or berries in moderation. Fill the cake molds, and place them in the oven. Bake for 15-20 min.

Almond Cookies

Ingredients

2 cups almond flour

1/2 cup erythritol

1/4 cup butter

2 chicken eggs

1 tsp extract of vanilla

1 tsp cinnamon

salt

halves of almonds

Cooking time: 30 min

Serves: 2-4

Calories per person: 496-992

Nutritional facts: total fat 18g, cholesterol 31mg, sodium 145mg, total carbohydrate 12g, protein 12 g

Directions

1. Preheat the oven to 355 °F.

2. While the oven is heating, mix almond flour, erythritol, cinnamon, and a pinch of salt in a bowl.

3. Beat the eggs in a small bowl. Add butter and vanilla. Stir.

4. Mix the dry ingredients with the egg mixture until evenly combined.

5. Form dough into small circles using a spoon.

6. Decorate circles with half an almond.

7. Line a baking sheet with parchment paper coated in butter. Put the cookies on it.

8. Bake for 10-15 min.

Carrot Nut Cake

Ingredients

50 g almond flour

25 g coconut flour

2 tbsp baking powder

50 g pecan

15 g chia seeds

100 g grated carrot

4 chicken eggs

100 g Philadelphia cream cheese

100 g sour cream (30%)

90 g butter

vanilla

cinnamon

salt

Cooking time: 1 h 10 min
Serves: 4
Calories per person: 520
Nutritional facts: total fat 46g, cholesterol 262mg, sodium 341mg, total carbohydrate 17g, protein 13g

Direction

1. Preheat oven to 320 °F.

2. Prepare the cream. In a blender, place the cream cheese, sour cream and vanilla to taste. Mix everything well until smooth. Allow the mixture to sit.

3. Mix almond and coconut flour, chia seeds and pecans. Add baking powder, salt, and cinnamon. Grind all these dry ingredients in the flour. You can leave large pieces.

4. Grated carrot.

5. Separate the yolks in the eggs. Beat the eggs white to add air. Mix the yolks.

6. Melt the butter and let cool. Mix the egg whites with the yolks. Add creamy melted butter. Mix again.

7. In the mixture add dry ingredients: mix flour, nuts and seeds. Gently stir manually or with a blender.

8. Fold the carrots evenly into the batter.

9. Place the batter onto a baking sheet and bake in the oven for 45 min.

10. Cool the cake and cut into several layers. Smear each layer with cream. Let the cake rest overnight in the refrigerator.

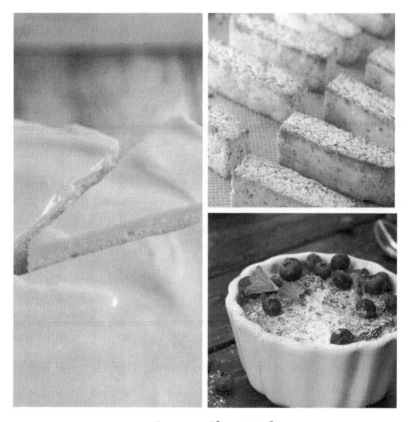

Lemon Cheesecake
Lemon Coconut Poppy Seeds Pie
Lemon and Blackberry Pudding

Lemon Cheesecake

Ingredients

200 g soft cream cheese

50 grams fatty cream

1 tbsp lemon juice

1 tsp stevia in liquid form

1 tsp lemon peel

Vanilla

Cooking time: 10 min + time for chilling
Serves: 3
Calories per person: 270

Nutritional facts: total fat 26.8g, cholesterol 81mg, sodium 207mg, total carbohydrate 2.7g, protein 5.6g

Directions

1. Put cream cheese and cream on a bowl Mix them with a mixer until uniform mass.

2. Add stevia, lemon juice, vanilla, lemon zest. Mix well.

3. Put the mixture into tart pans You may consume immediately. For best results, chill in the refrigerator for two hours to harden.

Lemon Coconut Poppy Seeds Pie

Ingredients
60 g coconut flour
4 chicken eggs
100 ml unsweetened natural yogurt
50 g coconut oil
2 tbsp coconut flakes
2 tsp baking powder
1 tsp vanilla powder
1 lemon
2 tbsp poppy

Cooking time: 40 min
Serves: 3
Calories per person: 603

Nutritional facts: total fat 46.8g, cholesterol 534mg, sodium 341mg, total carbohydrate 24.3g, protein 24.7g

Directions
1. Preheat oven to 345 °F.
2. Break the eggs. Add coconut flour, melted coconut oil, yogurt, vanilla powder, and baking powder. Stir all

ingredients until smooth. Let the dough rest for five min.

3. Wash and peel the lemon. Then cut off the top layer of peel and chop it in a blender. Juice lemon and add juice to the mixture, with crushed zest, and mix.

4. Prepare a mold with detachable edges. Line it with parchment paper and grease with coconut oil. Place dough on paper. Decorate the top of the cake with coconut flakes and poppy seeds. Bake for 25-30 min.

☐

Lemon and Blackberry Pudding

Ingredients
¼ cup coconut flour
5 chicken eggs
2 tbsp butter
2 tbsp coconut oil
2 tbsp oily cream
2 tbsp erythritol
one lemon
2 tsp lemon juice
1/2 cup blackberries
1/4 tsp baking powder
10 drops liquid stevia

Cooking time: 30-35 min
Serves: 4
Calories per person: 177

Nutritional facts: total fat 13.9g, cholesterol 16mg, sodium 86mg, total carbohydrate 16g, protein 5.9g

Directions
1. Preheat oven to 345 °F.

2. Separate egg yolks from whites. Whisk the yolks to a pale yellow color. Add erythritol and stevia and mix until evenly combined.

3. Add fatty cream, coconut oil, and lemon juice.

4. Wash and zest the lemon. Add zest to the mixture and mix.

5. Add the coconut flour and baking powder. Mix all the ingredients.

6. Add the blackberry to the mixture. Press the berries into it a little.

7. Bake pudding for 20-25 min. in the baking cups.

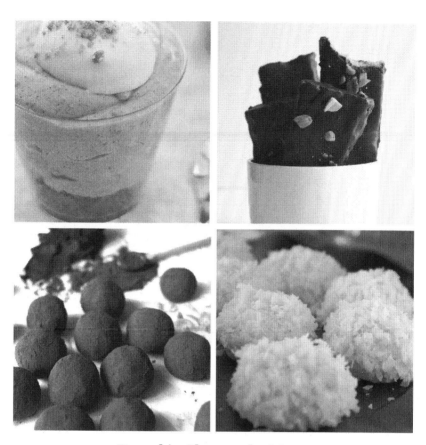

Pumpkin Cheesecake Mousse
Vegan Chocolate Turron
Vegan Chocolate Orange Truffles
Coconut Snowballs

Pumpkin Cheesecake Mousse

Ingredients
340 g softened cream cheese
420 g unsweetened pumpkin puree
½ cup erythritol
2 tsp pure vanilla extract
2 tbsp pumpkin pie spice
¾ cup heavy cream

Cooking time: 10 min + time for refrigerating
Serves: 10
Calories per person: 173

Nutritional facts: total fat 15.3g, cholesterol 50mg, sodium 108mg, total carbohydrate 17.9g, protein 3.5g

Directions
1. In a large mixing bowl, combine the cream cheese and pumpkin puree by hand. The mixture must be creamy, smooth, and without clumps.

2. Add vanilla, spices, erythritol, and heavy cream to the pumpkin mixture. Combine well.

3. Refrigerate mousse before serving.

Vegan Chocolate Turron

Ingredients
255   g dark chopped chocolate
2 tbsp melted coconut oil
40 g unsalted raw hazelnuts

Cooking time: 15 min + time for chill
Serves: 16
Calories per person: 106

Nutritional facts: total fat 8.3g, cholesterol 1mg, sodium 6mg, total carbohydrate 10.4g, protein 1.2g

Directions
1. Place dark chocolate in a saucepan. Cook over medium heat, stirring occasionally until chocolate is melted.

2. Remove chocolate from the heat. Add hazelnuts, and combine well.

3. Pour the chocolate-hazelnuts mixture into lined rectangular dish.

4. Cool to room temperature. Chop the turron.

5. If it's too hot in the room, keep turron in the fridge.

Vegan Chocolate Orange Truffles

Ingredients

200   pitted dates

50 g almond meal

2 tbsp unsweetened cocoa powder

Extra cocoa powder (for rolling the balls)

2 tbsp orange juice

Zest of 1 lemon

Cooking time: 10 min
Serves: 16
Calories per person: 52

Nutritional facts: total fat 1.7g, cholesterol 0mg, sodium 0mg, total carbohydrate 9.6g, protein 1.1g

Directions

1. Place pitted dates, almond meal, cocoa powder, orange juice, and lemon zest in a food processor or a powerful blender. Mix well.

2. Make the mixture into balls using your hands. Make 16 truffles.

3. Roll the candies in cocoa powder to taste.

Coconut Snowballs

Ingredients

95 g shredded coconut

35 g almond flour

80 g agave syrup

Cooking time: 10 min
Serves: 10
Calories per person: 65

Nutritional facts: total fat 3.7g, cholesterol 0mg, sodium 8mg, total carbohydrate 8.4g, protein 0.5g

Directions

1. Mix 75 g shredded coconut, flour, and syrup in a food processor until well combined.

2. Make 10 balls using your hands.

3. Roll the balls in 20 g shredded coconut.

4. You can keep these balls in a sealed container in a fridge for one week.

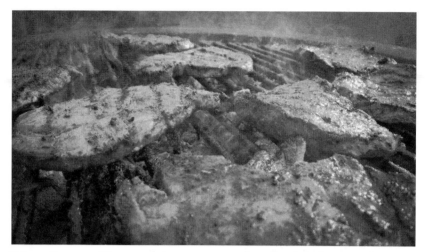

The keto diet recipe uses foods high in fats and proteins. In this case, carbohydrates should be completely excluded from the diet or at least reduced to a minimum. Originally, the keto diet was developed for people with epilepsy and obesity. Now, it is actively used among athletes who want tone their bodies to perfection. In addition, the ketogenic diet is used by women who dream of a more refined figure their figure without much physical exertion.

With the ketogenic diet, fats become the body's main source of energy. The diet can include any type of fat, but carbohydrates are reduced to zero. As you know, carbohydrates enter the body and are processed into glucose. Glucose is very important for brain function and is the brain's main fuel. In the absence of carbohydrates and, accordingly, glucose, the body looks for an alternative source of brain nutrition. This is fats, which the body converts into fatty acids and ketone bodies.

Ketone bodies are a separate group of metabolic products. They are formed in the liver. The main types are acetone, acetoacetic acid and beta-butoxybutyric acid. In the keto diet, ketone bodies are the main source of energy for the brain. Under the diet conditions, the body itself enters a special state: ketosis. In ketosis, the body is tuned to constantly split fats to obtain ketone bodies. With the keto diet, a person actively consumes fats, but also actively loses them, providing energy to the brain.

Who Is Suitable for Keto Diet?

The ketogenic diet is effective for rapid weight loss, when you need to reduce extra pounds in a short period of time. Such a diet can easily control appetite and let you forget about feeling hungry for a long time. In addition, it is used during the "drying" of athletes.

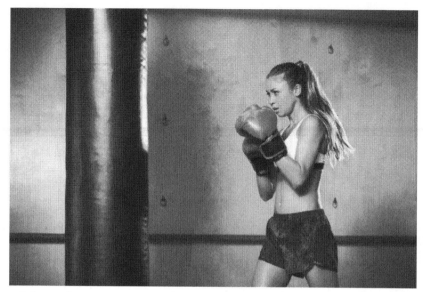

This diet is contraindicated for people with gastrointestinal disease, with any type of diabetes, with liver and kidney disease, during pregnancy and lactation, when working in severe and dangerous conditions, or for people who are engaged in mental work. In addition, it is not suitable for athletes who want to gain muscle mass.

Before the start of a ketogenic diet, it is absolutely necessary to consult a doctor. The specialist will determine whether your diet suits you and your body. □

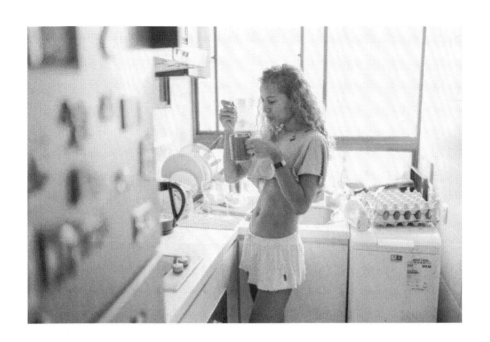

Uses and Harms

The most important advantage of a ketogenic diet is the ability to shed an impressive amount of excess weight in a very short time. For example, in two weeks it is quite possible to lose ten kilograms. In this case, a person loses only fat: muscle mass remains. However, there are a number of dangers that hide behind the impressive effectiveness.

PROS
- <u>Effective weight loss</u>

The diet allows you to get rid of subcutaneous fat
- <u>Cellulite loss</u>

The diet will eliminate the orange peel look on the buttocks and legs
- <u>No hunger</u>

During the diet, there is no feeling of hunger. After entering the state of ketosis, a person feels full.

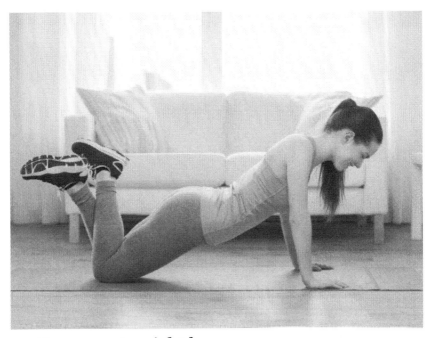

- <u>Permanent weight loss</u>

After the diet is over, the weight does not return for a long time. The body gets used to the constant intake of fats and does not see the need to store them.

- <u>Preservation of muscle mass</u>

During the diet, only fat is removed. Muscle mass remains untouched

- <u>A varied and nutritious menu</u>

The basis of a ketogenic diet is fats. A person can afford to eat rich foods.

- <u>A large selection of products</u>

On the keto diet, you do not have to starve yourself. Most food products remain available.

- Prevention of diabetes

The established diet helps reduce blood sugar, which is an effective means of preventing diabetes.

- Lower blood pressure

The keto diet normalize blood pressure better than other diets.

- Improved skin condition

Due to the decreased amount of carbohydrates consumed, the transition to a ketogenic diet is accompanied by an improvement in skin condition

☐

CONS

- Poor health in the first days of the diet

The body will consume glucose. During this period, a person suffers from terrible hunger and dizziness and, feels a decline in strength

- Brain function adversely affected

Carbohydrate starvation can reduce concentration and learning ability and increase memory loss. Prolonged carbohydrate deficiency can lead to irreversible changes

- Poisoning the body with toxic substances

The symptoms of which are manifested by the acetone odor of secretions

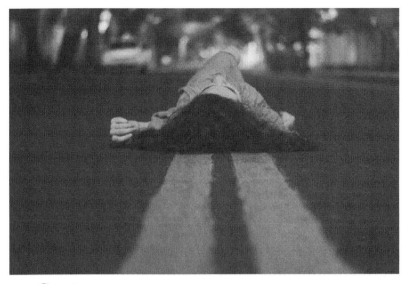

- Gout

The diet can cause gout because of increased meat dishes

- Constipation

Lack of fiber can provoke constipation and inflammation in the large intestine.

- Increased cholesterol

This problem can appear when eating saturated fats.

- Possible vitamin deficiency

Abandoning carbohydrates can lead to a deficiency of minerals and vitamins in the body.

- Possible discomfort

In the presence of gallstones, discomfort may occur.

- Other possible side effects

Seizures, hair loss, itching.

Basis of Keto Diets

The basis of the diet is a calorie deficit and an exact percentage compliance of consumed products. You can see it in our keto diet cookbook. Before starting the diet, you will need a calculator to calculate the number of Calories/person consumed per day and create your specific diet. The number of Calories/person consumed must be minimized. In addition, consider a regime that burns 300-500 kilocalories/person more than the body receives.

The formula for the keto diet is simple: 70% fats, 25% proteins, 5% green vegetables, 0% sugar and starch. That is, the foundation of the diet is fats, which should be about three quarters of your consumed products. Next are proteins. You should consume three times less protein than you consume fat. At first, the amount of proteins may be slightly larger, which can help you avoid poor health and stress. However, over time, the ratio should change in favor of fats.

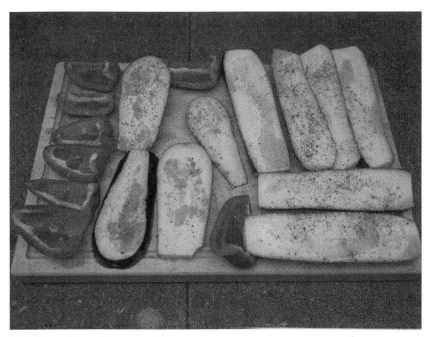

With the keto diet, you can eat a few green vegetables, but sugar and starch should be completely eliminated. At first, you may consume carbohydrates, but not more than 100 grams per day. With more than 100 grams of carbohydrates per day, the body does not go into ketosis.

Beginning and ending the diet should be gradual, first increase the amount of fat, and then slowly reduce it. For proteins, to begin, you can consume a larger portion (up to 45% per day), then slowly reduce this amount, and then gradually increase again. After carbohydrate fasting, you can-not begin to consume carbohydrates quickly. At the end of the diet, it is necessary to increase the share of carbohydrates by no more than 30 grams per day. Our book will be helpful as the keto diet for beginners.

How Do We Use the Keto Diet?

The transition to a ketogenic diet is divided into several stages.

The first stage lasts from eight to twelve hours. In this stage, the body will completely consume the available glucose reserves. During this time, a person feels quite normal. A little carbohydrate hunger may begin to appear, it is not strong and quite tolerable.

The second stage of keto diet lasts from one to three days. At this time, the body consumes glycogen reserves, which are contained in the liver and muscles. This is the most difficult period of a diet. A person feels hungry even with a stuffed stomach and, is constantly thinks of sweets; sweating and salivating increases; the stomach and liver begin to ache; nausea, dizziness, fatigue, and irritability occurs; and increased susceptibility to smells. This hunger can-not be satisfied even consuming in an unlimited amount of fats and proteins.

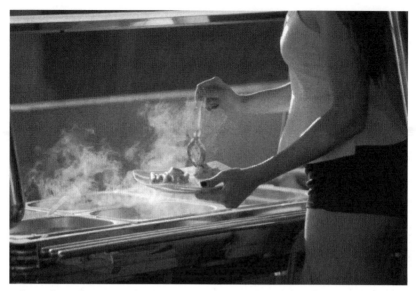

The third stage lasts a week. In the body, metabolism reorganization begins to occur as the body looks for an alternative to carbohydrates in fatty acids and proteins, including those contained in muscle mass. During this period, a person loses muscle tissue.

The fourth stages begins on the seventh day. The human body has learned to tolerate the lack of carbohydrates and switches to splitting available compounds. Here begins the splitting of fats and their transformation into ketone bodies. The body enters a state of ketosis. External signs of this condition are a specific acetone smell of the body, a lack of hunger, fatigue and dizziness.

Products for Keto Diet

For those who want to lose weight, the ketogenic diet has a large selection of products. While on this diet, you do not need to limit yourself to water and greens, but some products will still be off limits. A lot of them you will find in our simple keto recipes.

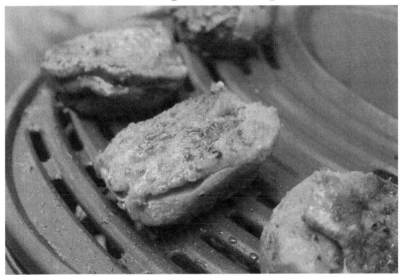

Allowed Products, Drinks and Seasonings

Meat products

Chicken, turkey, pork, beef, lamb, goat, and venison. You can even eat chicken skins.

Meat by-products

Liver, heart, and kidneys

Fish and seafood

Salmon, herring, shrimp, and squid. You can eat other fatty fish, but without breading

Saturated fats

Chicken, duck, goose fat

Eggs

Chicken and quail

Dairy products

Butter, sour cream, fatty cheeses, cottage cheese, and cream.

Oils

Creamy, olive, and coconut

Nuts

Brazilian, macadamia, pecans, walnuts, hazelnuts, and almonds

Seeds

Linseed, hemp, and chia

Vegetables

Leafy greens (spinach, lettuce, and green onions), cabbage, kohlrabi, broccoli, radish, celery, asparagus, cucumber, zucchini, bamboo shoots, beets, cherry tomatoes, and bell peppers.

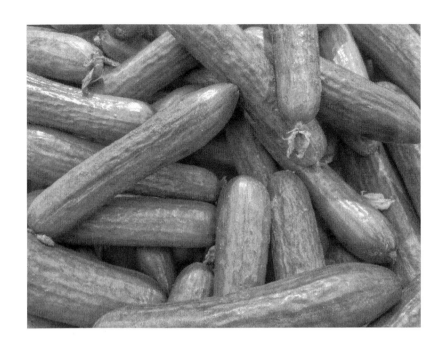

Fruit

Avocado

Berries

Blackberries, blueberries, strawberries, raspberries, and cranberries. You can eat berries in very limited quantities.

Beverages

Water, coffee (with cream or coconut milk), and tea (black, green).

Seasonings

Mayonnaise, mustard, salt, pepper, all spices and herbs, and lemon and lime juices.

Alcohol

Dry red wine, dry white wine, and unsweetened spirits. Although alcohol is allowed, it is better to abstain when on the keto diet.

You can take vitamins, which supplement trace elements in the body. In addition, pay special attention to water intake. When on a ketogenic diet, it is necessary to consume 2 to 3 liters of water. This will reduce the burden on the kidneys.

Prohibited Products, Drinks, and Seasonings

• All types of grains: wheat, rye, oats, corn, barley, millet, bulgur, sorghum, rice, amaranth, buckwheat, and sprouted grains.
• Products made from grains: flour, pasta, all kinds of pastries, bread, biscuits, pies, pizza, crackers, and breading.
• Legumes: soybeans, beans, and peas.
• Sugar and sweets: table sugar, corn syrup, agave syrup, ice cream, cakes, sweet puddings, and sweet soft drinks.
• Artificial sweeteners: aspartame, acesulfame, sucralose, and saccharin.

- Meat: pork with a high content of omega-6 fatty acids.
- Fish: high in omega-6 fatty acids.
- Dairy products: milk, margarine, cheese.
- Refined oils: sunflower, safflower, cottonseed, rape, and corn.
- Vegetables: potatoes, tomatoes, and carrots.
- Fruits: pineapples, mangoes, bananas, mandarin oranges, grapes, papayas, apples, pears, and kiwis.
- Dried fruits: raisins, prunes, dates, apricots, figs, and cherries.
- Beverages: fruit juices, sweet tea and coffee, and sweet soda water.
- Condiments: ketchup and sugar.
- Alcohol: beer, sweet wine, and cocktails.

When on the ketogenic diet, it is necessary to exclude all processed foods that contain carrageenan, sodium glutamate, sulfites, bisphenol A, and wheat gluten.

TIP! If you can-not do without a piece of bread in your diet, then you can bake bread from sesame, almond and coca flour. These types of flour are permitted while on a ketogenic diet. They can also be used for breading.

Preparing Keto Food

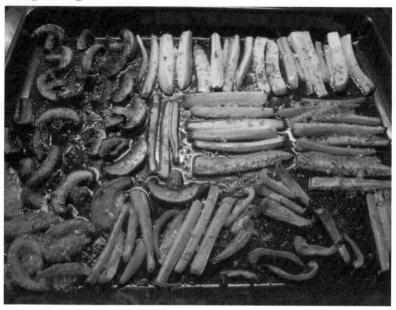

The developers of the ketogenic diet did not set limits and did not restrict cooking methods. On a keto diet, a person can do the following:

- Fry foods in oil or fat: meat, fish, seafood, and eggs
- Fry food over an open fire: meat, fish, and seafood
- Cooking on the grill: meat, fish
- Bake in the oven: meat, fish
- Boil: meat, eggs
- Stew: vegetables
- Steam: vegetables.